EVERYTHING ABOUT CERVICAL CANCER NUTRITION

Comprehensive Guide To Squamous Cell Carcinoma, Optimal Diet Plans, Superfoods, Key Nutrients For Prevention And Recovery

WALTON USELTON

DISCLAIMER

The content in this book is based on the author's expertise and understanding of food and nutrition. The author is not linked or associated with any corporation, business, or person. This book is designed for informative purposes only and should not be interpreted as professional medical advice. Readers should get medical advice before making any changes to their diet or lifestyle. The author takes no responsibility or liability for any repercussions arising from the use of the information included in this book.

Table of Contents

ABOUT THIS BOOK

"Cervical Cancer Nutrition" is more than just another book on healthy food; it's a complete guide designed exclusively for those dealing with cervical cancer. At its heart, this book is a source of information, shedding light on the complex link between diet and cervical cancer prevention and treatment.

The introduction guides readers through the process of learning about cervical cancer, from its terminology to its numerous kinds and the essential risk factors linked with it. Nutrition has an important role in both prevention and management. By emphasizing the significance of dietary choices in fighting this condition, the book lays the groundwork for the next chapters.

Chapter 1 looks into the fundamentals of nutrition, providing readers with critical information on macronutrients, micronutrients, and the importance of a well-balanced diet.

This chapter acts as a compass, directing readers towards healthy eating habits by interpreting nutrition labels and learning portion management and meal planning techniques.

Chapter 2 focuses on nutritional suggestions for cervical cancer prevention, with an emphasis on antioxidants, vitamins, and other micronutrients renowned for their powerful cancer-fighting qualities. Readers obtain essential insights for designing a diet fortified against cervical cancer by delving deeply into dietary fiber, folate, and phytonutrients.

Chapter 3 makes navigating the stormy seas of cancer treatment easier since it provides practical guidance on how to alleviate treatment-related side effects through a good diet. This chapter acts as a beacon of support for those enduring cancer treatment, covering everything from nausea management to hydration and adding protein-rich diets for tissue healing.

Maintaining a healthy weight emerges as a significant component of cervical cancer care in Chapter 4, where readers are equipped with weight management methods and the value of physical exercise. Readers gain confidence in this element of their health journey by practicing mindful eating and following the advice of healthcare specialists.

Chapter 5 takes readers on a journey to create a nutrient-dense food plan, emphasizing the need for customized meal plans based on individual requirements. Readers will learn how to include a variety of fruits and vegetables, as well as how to choose lean protein sources and good fats, to maintain a satisfying diet.

Chapter 6 focuses on cooking and food safety, teaching readers the necessity of appropriate food handling and storage, as well as healthy cooking techniques and meal prep procedures. With this information, readers can easily traverse the culinary environment, even if they have a hectic schedule or are eating out.

Chapter 7 emphasizes the emotional and social aspects of nutrition, encouraging readers to investigate coping techniques for emotional eating as well as the significance of obtaining social support. Readers develop a comprehensive approach to well-being by engaging in mindfulness activities and finding delight in healthful meals.

Chapter 8 delves into the world of supplements and herbal medicines, providing a balanced view of their possible advantages and hazards. This chapter emphasizes the necessity of talking with healthcare practitioners before including supplements in one's dietary plan, empowering readers to make educated health choices.

Long-term dietary solutions take priority in Chapter 9, which walks readers through the transition to a post-treatment diet and emphasizes the significance of frequent check-ups and screenings. By recognizing milestones and keeping inspired, readers are encouraged to continue good behaviors for long-term fitness.

The last chapter provides readers with a wealth of information and additional support networks, ranging from suggested reading and websites to support groups and local sources for fresh, healthful meals. Readers are empowered to continue their path toward optimum health and well-being by connecting with others and remaining informed.

INTRODUCTION

Definition And Types

Cervical cancer is a form of cancer that develops in the cells of the cervix, which is the bottom section of the uterus connected to the vagina. The cervix is an important part of delivery, and its cells may alter, leading to malignant development. Cervical cancer is classified into numerous forms, the most frequent of which are squamous cell carcinoma and adenocarcinoma. Squamous cell carcinoma originates from the flat, thin cells that line the outer surface of the cervix, while adenocarcinoma grows from the cervix's glandular cells.

Risk Factors

Several factors may raise the chance of acquiring cervical cancer. Infection with some strains of the human papillomavirus (HPV), which is transmitted sexually, is a major risk factor. Other risk factors include smoking, a weaker immune system, early sexual activity, several sexual partners, a history of sexually transmitted diseases, prolonged use of oral contraception, and a family history of cervical cancer.

Importance Of Nutrition In Prevention And Management

Nutrition is essential in the prevention and treatment of cervical cancer. A well-balanced diet rich in fruits, vegetables, whole grains, lean proteins, and healthy fats may improve general health and boost the immune system. Certain nutrients, such as antioxidants, vitamins, and minerals, have been related to a lower risk of cervical cancer, and they may also assist improve treatment results and lessen side effects.

An Overview Of The Book's Purpose

The goal of this book is to give complete information on nutrition's involvement in cervical cancer prevention and therapy. It will cover a wide range of nutrition topics, including dietary guidelines, particular nutrients of interest, and practical strategies for implementing good eating habits into everyday living. In addition, the book will look at the most recent research results and evidence-based dietary methods to help prevent and cure cervical cancer.

Who Is This Book For?

This book is aimed at anybody who wants to learn more about the role of diet in cervical cancer prevention and treatment. It is appropriate for patients with cervical cancer, their carers, healthcare professionals, nutritionists, dietitians, and anybody looking for accurate information on how food and nutrition affect cervical cancer risk and results. Whether you want to lower your chance of acquiring cervical cancer, assist someone going through treatment, or improve your nutritional intake for better health, this book will give you vital insights and practical advice to help you on your path.

CHAPTER ONE

Basics Of Nutrition

Essential Nutrients For Overall Health

Essential nutrients are the building blocks of a healthy organism, necessary for appropriate function and wellness. These nutrients include carbs, proteins, lipids, vitamins, minerals, and water. Carbohydrates give energy, proteins construct and repair tissues, lipids promote cell development and hormone synthesis, vitamins and minerals control a variety of body activities, and water keeps us hydrated and promotes digestion. Maintaining good health requires a sufficient consumption of these nutrients.

Foods containing carbohydrates include bread, pasta, rice, and fruits. They are the body's major source of energy, powering everyday activities and exercise.

Protein, on the other hand, is plentiful in foods such as meat, poultry, fish, beans, and nuts. They serve an important role in tissue development and repair, making them necessary for muscle growth and recovery.

Fats are often misunderstood, although they are essential for good health. Avocados, almonds, seeds, and olive oil provide healthful fats. These fats promote cell development, organ protection, and nutrient absorption. It is important to pick healthy fats over the bad ones found in processed and fried meals.

Vitamins and minerals are micronutrients that are needed in lower quantities but are as vital. They assist control of a variety of biological activities, including metabolism, immunological function, and bone health. Fruits, vegetables, complete grains, and lean meats are rich in vitamins and minerals.

Water is frequently disregarded, although it is critical for life. It maintains body temperature, distributes nutrients and wastes, and lubricates joints. Aim for at least eight glasses of water every day to keep hydrated and support body processes.

Understanding Macronutrients And Micronutrients

Macronutrients are nutrients that give energy and are required in big amounts. They consist of carbs, proteins, and lipids. These macronutrients are necessary for the body's energy production, tissue repair, and function regulation. Understanding the importance of each macronutrient might help you make more educated dietary choices.

Carbohydrates are the body's main source of energy. They are converted into glucose, which feeds our cells and provides energy for physical activities. Complex carbs, found in whole grains, fruits, and vegetables, are favored over simple carbohydrates, such as sugar and refined grains since they give long-term energy and vital nutrients.

Proteins are the fundamental building blocks of life, essential for tissue formation and repair. They are made up of amino acids, some of which are required and must be supplied from food. Animal proteins, such as meat, fish, and dairy, provide all required amino acids, while plant proteins, such as beans, lentils, and tofu, may be combined to create complete proteins.

Fats provide energy and are required for the absorption of fat-soluble vitamins as well as the maintenance of cell structure. Healthy fats, such as avocados, almonds, and olive oil, should be preferred over bad fats found in processed and fried meals. Fats should be taken in moderation since they are high in calories and, if ingested in excess, may lead to weight gain.

Micronutrients, on the other hand, are nutrients that are needed in lesser amounts but are still essential for general health. They include vitamins and minerals, which are needed for a variety of body activities such as metabolism, immunological function, and bone health. Fruits, vegetables, whole grains, and lean meats are rich in micronutrients.

Importance Of A Balanced Diet

A well-balanced diet is crucial for good health. It gives the body the nutrition it needs to operate correctly, keep energy levels stable, and avoid chronic disorders. A balanced diet includes a wide range of foods from all dietary categories, such as fruits, vegetables, whole grains, lean protein, and healthy fats.

Fruits and vegetables are high in vitamins, minerals, and antioxidants, which help the body fight illness and maintain general health.

Fill half of your plate with fruits and vegetables at each meal to ensure you receive enough of these important nutrients.

Whole grains, such as brown rice, quinoa, and oats, are high in fiber, which assists digestion and keeps you full and content. Choose whole grains over processed grains, such as white rice and white bread, which have lost their nutrients and fiber after processing.

Lean proteins such as chicken, fish, tofu, and lentils help to develop and repair tissues, as well as stimulate muscle growth and recovery. To decrease your saturated fat consumption, keep portion sizes in check and go for lean kinds of meat.

Avocados, almonds, seeds, and olive oil include healthy fats, which are necessary for heart health and cognitive function. Incorporate these fats into your diet in moderation to gain their advantages while avoiding unnecessary calories.

Reading Nutritional Labels

Nutrition labels give useful information regarding the nutritional composition of items, allowing you to make more educated eating decisions. Understanding how to read nutrition labels will allow you to choose items that meet your health objectives and dietary requirements.

Begin by looking at the serving size, which specifies how much food is used to calculate nutrition information. Keep track of the number of servings in each container and the calories per serving. This may help you control your portion sizes and monitor your calorie consumption.

Next, look at the macronutrient composition, which includes the quantity of carbs, proteins, and fats. Choose meals that are low in saturated and trans fats, cholesterol, and salt, yet abundant in fiber, vitamins, and minerals.

Check the ingredient list to discover what's in the meal. Ingredients are presented in decreasing order of weight, thus the first few ingredients account for the bulk of the product. Avoid items with a lengthy list of ingredients, particularly those with added sugars, artificial flavors, and preservatives.

Pay heed to any health or nutritional content claims on the package. While these statements might be informative, it's important to assess the whole nutritional profile of the product and how it fits into your overall diet.

Reading nutrition labels allows you to make educated food choices that match your nutritional requirements while also supporting your health objectives.

Portion Control And Meal Planning

Portion management is essential for keeping a healthy weight and avoiding overeating. It entails being careful of the quantity of food you consume and paying attention to your body's hunger and fullness signals. Meal planning may help you manage your portion sizes and make better food choices throughout the week.

Begin by using smaller dishes and bowls to better regulate portion amounts. Fill half of your plate with fruits and vegetables, a quarter with lean protein, and the remaining quarter with nutritious grains or starchy veggies. This balanced approach guarantees that you acquire a wide range of nutrients while keeping your calorie consumption under control.

Mindful eating entails paying attention to your body's hunger and fullness signals. Eat gently, savoring each meal, and stop when you're content, not excessively full. Avoid distractions like watching TV or going through your phone while eating since these may lead to mindless eating and overconsumption.

Meal planning is preparing meals and snacks in advance to ensure that you have healthy alternatives accessible throughout the week. Begin by establishing a weekly meal and snack plan based on your schedule and nutritional preferences. Choose meals that are healthful, simple to make, and can be prepared in bulk to save time.

Set aside time every week to do food shopping and prepare items for meals and snacks. To make healthy eating more easy, chop veggies, prepare grains and meats, and pre-portion snacks. Store leftovers in meal-sized amounts for quick grab-and-go alternatives on busy days.

Portion management and meal planning may help you maintain a healthy weight, meet your nutritional requirements, and make better choices in general. You may enjoy tasty and healthy meals while encouraging maximum health and well-being by eating and preparing them mindfully.

CHAPTER TWO

Nutritional Guidelines For Cervical Cancer Prevention

Antioxidants And The Prevention Of Cell Damage

Antioxidants are essential for reducing cell damage, which is especially important in the prevention of cervical cancer. Understanding their function starts with comprehending the idea of oxidative stress. Oxidative stress arises when the body's free radicals and antioxidants are out of equilibrium. Free radicals are unstable chemicals that may harm cells and DNA, possibly leading to cancer growth. Antioxidants neutralize free radicals, lowering the risk of cell damage.

Incorporating antioxidant-rich foods into your diet may help prevent cervical cancer. These include berries, citrus fruits, and kiwi, which are high in vitamin C, a powerful antioxidant. Vegetables such as spinach, kale, and sweet potatoes are strong in vitamin A, another potent antioxidant. Nuts, seeds, and vegetable oils are high in vitamin E, which completes the triad of vitamins needed to prevent oxidative stress.

Foods High In Vitamins A, C, And E

Vitamins A, C, and E are vital for general health, but their antioxidant characteristics make them particularly useful in the prevention of cervical cancer. Vitamin A is essential for maintaining healthy skin and mucous membranes, which serve as protective barriers against infections such as human papillomavirus (HPV), a major risk factor for cervical cancer.

Furthermore, vitamin A promotes immunological function, which aids the body's defense against malignant cell proliferation.

Vitamin C, commonly known as ascorbic acid, is an antioxidant that strengthens the immune system and aids in the healing of damaged tissues. It is critical for collagen production, which is required for wound healing and connective tissue integrity. Furthermore, vitamin C improves the body's capacity to absorb iron, which is an essential nutrient for general health.

Vitamin E is a fat-soluble antioxidant that defends cell membranes against oxidative damage. It also affects immunological function and skin health. Consuming vitamin-rich meals such as colorful fruits and vegetables, nuts, seeds, and whole grains will help prevent cervical cancer.

The Importance Of Folate And B Vitamins

Folate, along with other B vitamins such as B6 and B12, is essential for DNA synthesis and repair. Adequate folate consumption is especially essential for women of reproductive age because it prevents neural tube abnormalities in unborn kids. However, folate may help prevent cervical cancer by promoting healthy cell division and lowering the chance of DNA damage, which can lead to malignant growth.

In addition to folate, B vitamins such as B6 and B12 are necessary for good health and well-being. Vitamin B6, or pyridoxine, is involved in over 100 enzyme events in the body, including metabolism and neurotransmitter production. Vitamin B12, or cobalamin, is essential for nerve function and red blood cell synthesis.

Including foods high in folate and other B vitamins in your diet, such as leafy greens, legumes, fortified grains, and lean meats, may help prevent cervical cancer and promote overall health.

Dietary Fibre And Digestive Health

Dietary fiber is a plant material that cannot be digested yet is essential for digestive health and general well-being. There are two kinds of dietary fiber: soluble and insoluble. Soluble fiber dissolves in water and creates a gel-like material in the digestive system, which aids in slowing digestion and regulating blood sugar levels. Insoluble fiber bulks up stool and encourages regular bowel movements, avoiding constipation and lowering the risk of colon cancer.

Dietary fiber is useful in the prevention of cervical cancer for a variety of reasons. First, it increases regularity, which aids in the effective elimination of toxins and waste from the body. Second, a high-fiber diet may reduce circulating estrogen levels, a hormone linked to an increased risk of cervical cancer. Finally, fiber-rich foods including fruits, vegetables, whole grains, and legumes are often nutrient-dense and low in calories, making them excellent options for maintaining a healthy weight, another factor in cancer prevention.

Phytonutrients And Cancer-Fighting Properties

Phytonutrients, also known as phytochemicals, are naturally occurring molecules found in plants that have been proven to improve human health. Many phytonutrients have strong antioxidant and anti-inflammatory qualities, making them effective partners in the battle against cancer, particularly cervical cancer.

Colorful fruits and vegetables such as berries, citrus fruits, and dark leafy greens contain a kind of phytonutrient known as flavonoids. These chemicals have been found to decrease cancer cell proliferation and reduce inflammation in the body. Another category, known as carotenoids, provides fruits and vegetables with their brilliant colors and has been associated with a decreased risk of many malignancies, including cervical carcinoma.

Cruciferous plants such as broccoli, cauliflower, and Brussels sprouts contain sulfur-containing chemicals called glucosinolates, which have been found to have anti-cancer potential. These chemicals may assist in detoxifying toxins and limit cancer cell development.

Incorporating a variety of phytonutrient-rich foods into your diet, such as fruits, vegetables, whole grains, nuts, seeds, and legumes, may offer a wide range of cancer-fighting substances to help prevent cervical cancer and improve overall health.

CHAPTER THREE

Nutrition During Cancer Treatment

Dealing With Side Effects Such As Nausea And Loss Of Appetite

Side effects of cancer therapy include nausea and lack of appetite. These symptoms might make it difficult to maintain sufficient nutrition, but there are ways to manage them.

One strategy is to eat little, frequent meals throughout the day rather than three big ones. This may help avoid nausea by preventing the stomach from getting overfull. Choosing bland, readily digested items such as crackers, rice, and bananas may also help to soothe the stomach and relieve nausea.

Another recommendation is to avoid strong odors and flavors since these might cause nausea in certain individuals. Individuals feeling nausea may find it easier to consume lukewarm or room-temperature items rather than heated ones.

Those experiencing appetite loss should concentrate on nutrient-dense meals to ensure they are receiving enough vitamins and minerals. Nuts, seeds, avocados, and yogurt are examples of foods that are high in nutrients yet have a tiny portion size.

In addition to dietary adjustments, medicines are available to alleviate nausea and increase appetite. It's critical to collaborate closely with a healthcare physician to determine the best mix of drugs and dietary practices to properly treat these adverse effects.

Importance Of Hydration

Staying hydrated is essential for general health, but it becomes even more important during cancer treatment.

Dehydration may exacerbate side effects such as weariness and nausea, thus it is critical to prioritize water during the treatment period.

Drinking water is the most effective approach to remain hydrated, although herbal tea, broth, and fruit juices may also help with fluid consumption. Caffeinated and alcoholic beverages should be avoided since they might dehydrate the body.

Some people may struggle to drink enough water, particularly if they have nausea or oral sores. In certain circumstances, sucking on ice chips or popsicles might assist boost fluid intake while minimizing pain.

Monitoring urine output may also be an effective approach to determine hydration status. Dark yellow urine may indicate dehydration, while light yellow or clear urine indicates proper hydration.

It is important to address any hydration difficulties with a healthcare practitioner, as they may provide tailored suggestions based on individual requirements and treatment regimens.

Protein-Rich Foods For Tissue Repair

Protein is vital for tissue regeneration and general health, making it especially critical for cancer patients. Including protein-rich meals in your diet may help the body repair and maintain muscular mass after therapy.

Lean meats, poultry, fish, eggs, dairy products, legumes, nuts, and seeds are all excellent protein sources. These foods provide important amino acids, which the body needs to form and repair tissues.

Individuals who have nausea or trouble swallowing may benefit from softer protein sources such as scrambled eggs, Greek yogurt, or protein drinks. These solutions may be simpler to digest and more appealing to folks who have sensitive stomachs.

In rare circumstances, a healthcare physician may offer protein supplements to guarantee appropriate consumption, particularly if dietary restrictions or side effects are limiting food intake. It is important to follow their recommendations and choose high-quality supplements that are suited to your specific requirements.

Easy-To-Digest Foods

During cancer treatment, it is critical to concentrate on meals that are simple to digest to reduce gastrointestinal pain and improve overall health. Choosing bland, low-fiber foods may assist in relieving digestive problems and make eating more pleasant.

Easy-to-digest meals include cooked vegetables without skins or seeds, white rice, simple spaghetti, bread, crackers, and applesauce.

These meals are mild on the digestive tract and are less likely to irritate or worsen current problems.

It's also important to watch your portion sizes, since eating huge meals may place extra pressure on the digestive system. Instead, strive for smaller, more frequent meals and snacks throughout the day to give a consistent supply of nutrients without overloading the stomach.

Individuals suffering from particular digestive difficulties, such as diarrhea or constipation, may need to make additional dietary changes to adequately control symptoms. Working with a healthcare physician or certified dietitian may help you create a personalized dietary plan that addresses these issues.

Supplements Role In Supporting Treatment

In addition to dietary adjustments, vitamins may aid in cancer therapy and general health. However, supplementing should be approached with caution and in consultation with a healthcare expert before adding any new items to the routine.

Some supplements that might be useful during cancer therapy include:

• Vitamin D promotes immunological function and bone health, especially during therapy.

• Omega-3 fatty acids may decrease inflammation and improve heart health.

• Probiotics may support a healthy gut microbiota and alleviate gastrointestinal symptoms like diarrhea.

- Multivitamins provide a complete combination of vitamins and minerals to address nutritional gaps in the diet.

It is important to choose supplements from trusted providers and adhere to suggested doses precisely. Excessive doses of some vitamins and minerals may be dangerous, so consult with a healthcare expert to identify the best supplementation strategy for your specific requirements.

Finally, diet is critical in helping cancer patients. Maintaining nutritional status and supporting general health during this difficult period may be accomplished by focusing on easy-to-digest meals, keeping hydrated, consuming protein-rich foods, and considering supplements as required. Working together with a healthcare professional or qualified dietitian may help you create a personalized nutrition plan that matches your specific requirements and maximizes treatment success.

CHAPTER FOUR

Maintaining A Healthy Weight

Understanding BMI And Its Significance

BMI, or Body Mass Index, is a useful measure that determines if a person is underweight, normal weight, overweight, or obese depending on their height and weight. It's a straightforward calculation: divide your weight in kilograms by your height in meters squared. Understanding your BMI might help you better understand your overall health and any weight-related problems.

Maintaining a healthy weight is critical for cervical cancer patients' overall health and treatment success. According to research, being overweight or obese increases the likelihood of getting cervical cancer and may influence treatment efficacy and recovery.

Conversely, being underweight might weaken the immune system and impair the body's capacity to combat cancer cells.

Understanding your BMI allows you to determine if you are in a healthy weight range or whether changes are needed to support your health journey. Healthcare specialists can assist analyze BMI readings and provide tailored suggestions for obtaining and maintaining a healthy weight.

Healthy Strategies For Weight Management

Achieving and maintaining a healthy weight requires making long-term lifestyle adjustments that improve overall well-being. Instead of relying on fad diets or drastic measures, aim to make modest, long-term improvements to your food patterns and physical activity levels.

Begin by adding more complete, nutrient-dense foods to your diet, such as fruits, vegetables, lean meats, and whole grains. These foods include critical vitamins, minerals, and antioxidants that help the immune system and general health. Fill your plate with a mix of colors and textures to ensure you acquire a wide range of nutrients.

In addition to eating correctly, make frequent physical exercise a priority in your weight control strategy. Exercise not only burns calories, but it also improves cardiovascular health, builds muscles, and elevates mood. Find activities you love, such as walking, swimming, yoga, or dancing, and commit to at least 150 minutes of moderate-intensity activity every week.

Importance Of Physical Activity

Physical exercise is important for maintaining a healthy weight and lowering the risk of chronic illnesses like cancer. Staying active may help people with cervical cancer improve their treatment results, reduce side effects, and improve their general quality of life.

Regular exercise has been demonstrated to improve immune function, decrease inflammation, and promote healthy circulation, all of which benefit cancer patients. Exercise may also assist with typical side effects of cancer therapy, such as tiredness, nausea, and depression, by generating endorphins and boosting mood.

To maximize the advantages of physical activity, include a combination of aerobic exercise, weight training, and flexibility exercises in your program. Begin cautiously, then progressively increase the intensity and length of your exercises as your fitness improves. Remember to listen to your body and check with your healthcare team before beginning any new fitness program, particularly when undergoing cancer treatment.

Mindful Eating Practices

Mindful eating entails paying close attention to your food choices, hunger signals, and eating patterns without judgment or distraction. It is about being more aware of your body's requirements and developing a pleasant connection with food.

Slow down during meals, savor each mouthful, and pay attention to your body's signals of hunger and fullness. Avoid eating in front of devices or when preoccupied, since this may lead to overeating and a detachment from your body's signals.

Choose meals that feed your body and please your taste senses, and try to eat with purpose rather than out of boredom, stress, or routine. Being more attentive to your eating habits allows you to make healthier choices, better manage your hunger, and have a more pleasant connection with food.

Seeking Help From Healthcare Professionals

Maintaining a healthy weight and implementing lifestyle adjustments may be difficult, particularly after a cancer diagnosis. That's why it's important to seek help from healthcare experts who can provide advice, encouragement, and personalized suggestions based on your specific requirements and circumstances.

Oncologists, nutritionists, physical therapists, and other experts may be part of your healthcare team and may provide guidance and support during your cancer treatment. Please do not hesitate to contact them if you need help with weight control, dietary counseling, exercise programming, or mental support.

In addition to professional advice, try attending support groups or interacting with others who have gone through similar circumstances.

Sharing your struggles, achievements, and insights with others helps foster a feeling of community and belonging, which can be quite powerful during tough times.

By actively interacting with your healthcare team and requesting assistance from others, you may negotiate the intricacies of weight control with confidence and resilience. Remember that you are not alone on this trip, and there are tools and support systems available to assist you along the road.

CHAPTER FIVE

Create A Nutrient-Rich Diet Plan

Creating A Personalized Meal Plan

Creating a personalized meal plan is the foundation of a healthy diet, particularly for individuals fighting cervical cancer. Individual dietary demands vary depending on age, weight, exercise level, and general health. Begin by speaking with a qualified dietitian or nutritionist, who can analyze your unique requirements and assist you in designing a meal plan that is personalized to your needs.

The method usually includes analyzing your current eating habits, detecting any deficiencies, and advising changes to ensure you get enough nutrients to support your health and recovery. Your meal plan should be practical and sustainable, taking into consideration your tastes, lifestyle, and any dietary constraints you may have.

Incorporating A Variety Of Fruits And Vegetables

Fruits and vegetables are nutritious powerhouses, including vitamins, minerals, antioxidants, and fiber, all of which are necessary for optimum health and well-being. To get the most out of your everyday diet, include a variety of fruits and vegetables.

To ensure you obtain a mix of nutrients, include leafy greens, berries, citrus fruits, cruciferous veggies, and root vegetables in your diet. Experiment with various cooking techniques, such as steaming, roasting, or stir-frying, to add diversity to your meals while also improving flavor and texture.

Choosing Lean Protein Sources

Protein is essential for maintaining and rebuilding bodily structures, boosting immunological function, and increasing satiety. When choosing protein sources for your diet, look for lean ones with minimal saturated fat and cholesterol.

Skinless chicken, fish, tofu, lentils, eggs, and low-fat dairy products are all excellent sources of lean protein. Including a variety of protein sources in your meals ensures that you get the full spectrum of important amino acids required for good health.

Healthy Fats For Brain And Heart Health

Despite their negative image, fats are an important part of a well-balanced diet because they provide energy and help in the absorption of fat-soluble vitamins.

However, not all fats are created equal.

Include healthy fats, such as avocados, nuts, seeds, olive oil, and fatty fish like salmon and trout. These fats include omega-3 fatty acids, which have been found to promote brain function, decrease inflammation, and lessen the risk of heart disease.

Limiting Processed And Sugary Foods

Processed and sugary foods have little nutritional value and may lead to weight gain, inflammation, and other health concerns, therefore they should be taken in moderation.

Instead, focus on full, nutrient-dense meals that fuel your body and promote general well-being. Choose whole grains, fresh fruits and vegetables, lean proteins, and healthy fats, while limiting your consumption of processed snacks, sugary drinks, and refined carbs.

By following these suggestions and tailoring your meal plan to your specific requirements, you can create a nutrient-dense diet that promotes your health and well-being while fighting cervical cancer. Remember to keep hydrated, listen to your body, and make any necessary modifications to ensure you feel your best every day.

CHAPTER SIX

Cooking And Food Safety

Importance Of Proper Food Handling And Storage

Proper food handling and storage are critical for lowering the risk of foodborne disease and preserving the nutritional value of your meals. When it comes to cervical cancer nutrition, food safety is critical for maintaining your entire health and well-being.

First and foremost, it is critical to recognize the significance of cleanliness throughout the food handling process. Washing your hands properly before and after handling food, as well as frequently cleaning surfaces and utensils, may help prevent the spread of hazardous germs. Additionally, separating raw meats from ready-to-eat meals and keeping them in separate containers or compartments in the refrigerator might help avoid cross-contamination.

When it comes to storage, appropriate temperature regulation is essential. Refrigerators should be set at 40°F (4°C) or lower to limit bacterial development, while freezers should be maintained at 0°F (-18°C) to retain frozen food quality. Keeping perishable foods chilled and kept in airtight containers may help to prolong their shelf life and avoid spoiling.

Healthy Cooking Methods

Using healthy cooking techniques is critical for retaining the nutritional content of meals while limiting your consumption of bad fat and calories. Individuals with cervical cancer should prioritize nutrition preservation and flavor improvement while cooking.

Steaming is one of the healthiest cooking techniques since it includes heating food over boiling water rather than immersing it. Steaming preserves natural vitamins and minerals in foods while keeping them soft and tasty. Another useful method is baking or roasting, which enables items to cook in their fluids while forming a delectable exterior crust. This approach is best suited for vegetables, lean meats, and fish.

Grilling is another popular cooking technique that imparts a smokey flavor to dishes without using excessive fats or oils. However, it is critical to avoid charring or blackening meats since this might produce toxic substances associated with cancer risk. To reduce carcinogen development, use low and moderate grilling rather than indirect heat.

Read Food Labels For Hidden Ingredients

Understanding how to understand food labels is vital for making educated eating decisions. When it comes to cervical cancer nutrition, identifying hidden elements such as added sugars, bad fats, and artificial additives is critical for keeping a balanced diet.

Begin by examining the ingredient list for any unknown or unpronounceable compounds, which are often synthetic additions or preservatives. Take note of the order in which the components are mentioned since manufacturers are obligated to report them in decreasing order of predominance by weight. The ingredients indicated at the beginning are in larger proportions than those listed at the end.

When analyzing food labels, take into account serving sizes and nutritional value per serving. When taken in excessive numbers, even ostensibly nutritious goods might contain significant levels of sugar, salt, or dangerous fats. Choose meals with little processing and elements you recognize to help you achieve your cervical cancer dietary objectives.

Meal Preparation Tips For Busy Schedules

Meal preparation is an effective approach for saving time and ensuring that healthy meals are always accessible, particularly for those who have hectic schedules. By devoting a part of your weekly time to meal planning, purchasing, and preparation, you can simplify your cooking process and make healthier choices throughout the week.

Begin by developing a meal plan that includes a range of nutrient-dense foods such as fruits, vegetables, whole grains, lean meats, and healthy fats. Choose dishes that can be easily prepared in big quantities and portioned for numerous meals. Invest in high-quality storage containers to keep prepared supplies and meals fresh for the whole week.

Strategies For Eating Out Healthy

Eating out may be difficult when attempting to maintain a healthy diet, but with the appropriate tactics, it is easy to make nutritious choices even while away from home. When managing cervical cancer nutrition, consider portion sizes, ingredients, and cooking techniques to help you navigate restaurant menus more successfully.

Begin by studying restaurant menus in advance and selecting restaurants that include healthy alternatives such as salads, grilled meats, and vegetable-based entrees. Look for customizable alternatives that let you make replacements or changes to meet your dietary needs or constraints.

When ordering, choose baked, grilled, steaming, or roasted over fried or breaded. To keep your consumption under control, order dressings, sauces, and condiments on the side, and prioritize whole meals like fruits, vegetables, and lean protein. Additionally, to minimize overeating, try splitting dinners or asking for a half quantity.

By using these healthy eating practices, you may enjoy restaurant meals without jeopardizing your cervical cancer nutrition objectives. With a little forethought and attention, you can make healthy choices that benefit your entire health and well-being, even while eating out.

CHAPTER SEVEN

The Emotional And Social Aspects Of Nutrition

Coping With Emotional Eating

Emotional eating may be a big difficulty for those with cervical cancer. It's important to recognize that emotions often impact our eating patterns, leading to overeating or selecting unhealthy meals. Coping with emotional eating entails being aware of your emotions and their relationship to food, as well as discovering alternate strategies to handle those feelings without turning to food.

One helpful technique is to maintain a food diary, documenting not only what you eat but also how you feel before and after eating. This might help you discover trends and causes of emotional eating. Furthermore, practicing mindfulness may help you become more aware of your body's hunger and fullness signals, helping you to differentiate between physical and emotional hunger.

Another beneficial strategy is to discover better methods to deal with stress and emotions, such as participating in physical exercise, practicing relaxation techniques like deep breathing or meditation, or obtaining assistance from friends, family, or a therapist. By creating a toolbox of alternative coping techniques, you may minimize your dependency on food to comfort your emotions.

Importance Of Social Support

Social support is essential in the treatment of cervical cancer, including nutritional factors. A strong support network may provide encouragement, accountability, and practical aid in making healthy eating choices and adhering to dietary guidelines. Whether it's friends, family, support groups, or healthcare experts, surrounding oneself with positive people may make a big impact on your nutritional journey.

Friends and family may assist by cooking healthful meals together, accompanying you to medical appointments, or just listening when you're feeling overwhelmed. Support groups may also be very beneficial for connecting with people who are going through similar situations, exchanging insights and resources, and finding unity in the pursuit of improved health.

Seeking Counselling Or Therapy As Needed

Coping with cervical cancer may trigger a broad variety of feelings, including fear, worry, grief, and anger. It is critical to recognize when these feelings become overpowering and seek professional assistance if required. Counseling or therapy may provide you with a safe place to explore and process your emotions, acquire coping methods, and build resilience in the face of hardship.

A therapist may work with you to address underlying problems that contribute to emotional eating, such as prior trauma or poor self-image, and help you develop a healthy connection with food and yourself. Furthermore, therapy may provide you with methods to manage stress, improve communication with loved ones, and improve your general emotional well-being, all of which are essential for maintaining a healthy lifestyle throughout cancer treatment.

Mindfulness Exercises For Stress Reduction

Mindfulness activities are effective strategies for stress reduction and general well-being. Mindfulness, which promotes present-moment awareness and nonjudgmental acceptance, may help you negotiate the difficulties of cervical cancer with more resilience and serenity. Incorporating mindfulness into your everyday routine may help you decrease stress, improve emotional control, and feel more connected to yourself and others.

Simple mindfulness techniques, including focused breathing, body scans, and mindful eating, may be incorporated into your daily routine to enhance relaxation and inner peace. Taking only a few minutes every day to stop, breathe, and ground yourself in the present moment may have a significant impact on your mental and emotional health, helping you to face difficulties with better clarity and serenity.

Finding Joy In Preparing And Consuming Nutritious Foods

Despite the difficulties of treating cervical cancer, finding delight in making and eating healthy meals may be both nourishing and enjoyable. Cooking can be a creative and soothing pastime, enabling you to express yourself, try new flavors, and take satisfaction in producing nutritious meals for yourself and your loved ones.

Include a range of colorful fruits, vegetables, whole grains, and lean meats in your meals to provide a well-balanced diet high in critical nutrients. Experiment with herbs, spices, and healthy cooking methods to improve the flavor and pleasure of your food. Also, remember to savor each mouthful attentively, paying attention to the flavors, textures, and sensations of eating.

By seeing cooking and eating as chances for self-care and sustenance, you may create a good connection with food and prioritize your health and well-being during your cancer treatment. Remember to be kind to yourself and enjoy minor triumphs along the road, since each healthy meal is a step towards healing and energy.

CHAPTER EIGHT

Supplements And Herbal Remedies

Common Supplements For Cancer Patients

Certain nutrients may help manage cervical cancer and improve general health. Some of the most widely suggested vitamins for cancer patients are:

1. Vitamin D: Vitamin D is required for bone health and immunological function. Patients with cervical cancer often have low levels of vitamin D, which may be rectified with supplementation.

2. Fish oil contains omega-3 fatty acids, which help decrease inflammation and improve heart health. They are also known to improve the effectiveness of chemotherapy.

3. Probiotics are helpful microorganisms that improve intestinal health. Probiotics may help relieve cancer-related side effects including diarrhea and other gastrointestinal disorders.

4. Vitamin C: Vitamin C, known for its immune-boosting effects, may help with general health and may increase the body's reaction to therapy.

5. B vitamins, notably B12, and folate, are essential for energy generation and cell maintenance, making them especially useful during cancer therapy.

Potential Benefits And Risks

While supplements may provide several advantages, they can pose hazards, particularly when used without competent counsel.

Benefits

- Correction of Nutrient Deficiencies in Cancer Patients: Poor appetite, nausea, and other treatment side effects may lead to nutritional deficiencies. Supplements may help address nutritional deficits.

• Vitamin C and probiotics may strengthen the immune system, aiding in fighting off infections and diseases.

• Omega-3 fatty acid supplements help decrease inflammation and discomfort, leading to improved quality of life.

Risks

• Certain supplements may interfere with chemotherapy and other cancer therapies, lowering their efficacy or producing unpleasant consequences. For example, excessive dosages of antioxidants such as vitamin E may impair the efficacy of radiation treatment.

• Excessive supplement use might cause toxicity. For example, high levels of vitamin D may produce hypercalcemia, which can lead to kidney stones and other health problems.

• Unproven Efficacy: Not all supplements are scientifically proven to be helpful. Some herbal medicines may not give the advantages claimed and might even be hazardous.

Herbal Remedies And Their Efficacy

Herbal medicines have been utilized for millennia in traditional medicine and are becoming popular among cancer patients. However, their efficiency varies, so approach them with care.

Common Herbal Remedies:

• Turmeric contains curcumin, which has anti-inflammatory and antioxidant benefits. According to certain research, it may assist in slowing the progression of cancer.

• Green Tea Extract: High in antioxidants, said to have cancer-fighting effects. Epigallocatechin gallate (EGCG), a chemical found in green tea, may help limit cancer cell proliferation.

• Ginger is often used to treat nausea caused by chemotherapy. Ginger also has anti-inflammatory effects.

• Milk Thistle may help promote liver health, especially for people undergoing chemotherapy.

• Echinacea is known to strengthen the immune system, although its usefulness in cancer patients is still being studied.

Evaluating Effectiveness

• Look for supplements supported by scientific research. For example, although some research suggests that turmeric has anti-cancer effects, further clinical trials are required to prove its usefulness.

- Assess study quality and size. Small or poorly planned research may not provide trustworthy results.

- Consult your healthcare professional before beginning any herbal medicine to confirm safety and compatibility with your treatment plan.

Before using supplements, consult with your healthcare provider.

Before beginning any supplement or herbal cure, consult with your healthcare physician. Here's how to handle this:

1. Create a list of all the vitamins and herbal therapies you're considering. Include information on doses and why they are taken.

2. Discuss Your Treatment Plan: Tell your healthcare practitioner about your current treatment plan, including any drugs you are taking. This allows them to examine possible interactions.

3. **Request advice:** Ask your healthcare professional for advice on safe and effective supplements based on your unique requirements and treatment plan.

4. **Follow Up Regularly:** Keep your healthcare practitioner informed of any new supplements you begin, and report any adverse effects or changes in your condition.

Carefully include supplements in your overall nutrition plan.

Supplements should be included in your entire dietary plan after careful evaluation and consultation with a healthcare practitioner.

Steps For Integration

1. **Assess Your Needs:** Determine which nutrients you may be missing based on your diet, treatment side effects, and general health. This may be accomplished using blood testing and nutritional evaluations.

2. Begin slowly, introducing one supplement at a time to evaluate its effects and minimize any unpleasant reactions.

3. **Balance with Food:** Remember that supplements are intended to enhance, not replace, your diet. Maintain a well-balanced diet that includes fruits and vegetables, lean meats, and whole grains.

4. **Monitor Your Progress:** Keep note of any changes in your health or symptoms after taking a new supplement. Adjust doses or cease usage as advised by your healthcare practitioner.

5. **Avoid mega-dosing:** Stick to the appropriate doses. More is not necessarily better, and taking too much of some vitamins might be dangerous.

By following these rules and communicating openly with your healthcare team, you may safely and successfully include vitamins and herbal medicines in your cervical cancer nutrition plan.

CHAPTER NINE

Long-Term Nutritional Strategy

Transitioning To The Post-Treatment Diet

Following cervical cancer treatment, shifting to a post-treatment diet is critical for recovery and long-term health. This phase requires careful consideration of dietary requirements to aid the body's healing process, restore energy levels, and avoid recurrence. Here are the stages for a good transition:

1. Reintroducing Nutrients Gradually:

• Add fruits, vegetables, whole grains, lean meats, and healthy fats to your diet. This ensures you get a variety of critical vitamins and minerals.

• For those experiencing nausea or appetite loss throughout therapy, start with modest, frequent meals to prevent overloading the digestive system.

2. Focus on Hydration:

• Proper fluid intake is crucial. Aim for at least 8-10 glasses of water every day to aid with toxin elimination and general body function.

• Include hydrating meals like cucumbers, melons, and soups.

3. Monitor Digestive Health:

• Observe how your body reacts to various meals. Some people may suffer sensitivities or intolerances after therapy.

• Probiotic-rich foods such as yogurt, kefir, and fermented vegetables may help reestablish healthy gut flora.

4. Seek professional guidance:

• Collaborate with an oncology-specialized dietitian or nutritionist to develop a personalized post-treatment nutrition plan.

• Regular visits may assist tailor your diet to your healing process and nutritional requirements.

The Need For Regular Check-Ups And Screenings

Regular check-ups and screenings are essential parts of long-term health care after cervical cancer therapy. These sessions assist in monitoring your recovery and spotting any symptoms of recurrence early on. Here's why they matter and what to expect:

1. Early detection of recurrence:

Regular pelvic examinations, Pap tests, and HPV testing may detect problems early, improving the likelihood of effective management.

• Regular imaging tests (e.g. CT scans or MRIs) may be advised to detect new growths.

2. Monitoring the Side Effects:

• Long-term adverse effects of treatments, such as lymphedema, bone density loss, or hormone abnormalities, may need continuing monitoring.

• Your healthcare practitioner may propose treatments and lifestyle changes to reduce these effects.

3. Nutritional assessments:

• Routine check-ups assess nutritional status to provide a balanced diet for optimal health.

• Blood testing may identify deficiencies that can be corrected with diet or supplements.

4. Personalised Health Plans:

• Your healthcare team may customize your follow-up treatment plan based on the findings of your check-up.

• The plan may include dietary changes, physical exercise suggestions, and stress/emotional management measures.

Keeping Healthy Habits For Long-Term Wellness

Adopting and sustaining healthy behaviors is essential for attaining long-term well-being after cervical cancer therapy. These practices promote general health, lower the chance of recurrence, and improve quality of life. Here are some practical strategies to develop these habits:

1. Balanced Diet:

• Increase your intake of fruits, vegetables, lean proteins, whole grains, and healthy fats. This supplies the nutrients required to maintain immunological function and general health.

• Avoid processed meals, sweets, and bad fats that may cause inflammation and health difficulties.

2. Regular Physical Activity:

• Perform at least 150 minutes of moderate aerobic or 75 minutes of strenuous activity each week, along with muscle-strengthening activities.

Walking, swimming, yoga, and strength exercises may boost cardiovascular health, improve mood, and help maintain a healthy weight.

3. Adequate Sleep:

• Get 7-9 hours of excellent sleep every night to promote bodily recovery and regeneration.

• establish a regular sleep schedule, avoid coffee and gadgets before bedtime, and establish a relaxing sleep environment.

4. Stress Management:

• Add stress-reducing activities to your routine, such as meditation, deep breathing exercises, or hobbies.

• Consider support groups or counseling to address emotional challenges after therapy.

Adjusting Dietary Needs Based On Changing Health Status

Your dietary requirements may alter over time, particularly when your health condition improves after therapy. It's critical to adapt your dietary strategy to match these shifting demands. Here are suggestions for successfully adapting your diet:

1. Regular Nutritional Reviews:

• Regularly meet with a nutritionist to examine and alter your diet depending on your health state and new medical discoveries.

• Keep a food journal to monitor your nutritional intake and find areas for improvement.

2. Incorporate Specific Nutrients.

• Adjust your nutritional intake based on your health requirements. For example, if you're concerned about bone density, eat calcium and vitamin D-rich foods like dairy, leafy greens, and fortified meals.

• To combat weariness, consume lean meats, legumes, and fortified cereals rich in iron and vitamin B12.

3. Adapt to physical changes.

• If you have difficulties swallowing or digesting specific meals, consider modifying their texture and preparation techniques.

• Soft meals, purees, and smoothies are healthy and easily digestible for persons with digestive difficulties.

4. Listen to your body.

• Be mindful of how various meals affect your mood. Certain foods may produce pain or bad reactions; modify your diet appropriately.

• Be open to testing new meals and dishes that align with your nutritional requirements and taste preferences.

Celebrating Milestones And Remaining Motivated

Celebrating accomplishments and keeping motivated is critical for sustaining a happy attitude and healthy behaviors. Here's how to make this trip fun and rewarding:

1. Set achievable goals:

• Organize your long-term health objectives into smaller, more doable milestones. This makes development seem more manageable and keeps you motivated.

• Celebrate minor achievements, such as adhering to a monthly workout plan or attempting a new healthy meal.

2. Reward yourself:

• Select incentives that support healthy behaviors. For example, reward yourself with new fitness gear, a peaceful spa day, or a fun culinary class.

• Non-food incentives may keep you focused on your health and well-being.

3. Stay connected:

• Participate in support groups or communities to connect with others going through similar situations. Sharing your journey and enjoying each other's triumphs may be motivating and inspiring.

• Connect with friends and family who support your healthy living choices.

4. Maintain a positive mindset:

• Prioritise accomplishments over setbacks. An optimistic mindset may boost your motivation and general well-being.

• Keep a thankfulness notebook to reflect on your accomplishments and health improvements.

By applying these methods, you may confidently traverse the post-treatment period, ensuring that you live a healthy, balanced lifestyle that promotes long-term well-being.

CHAPTER TEN

Long-Term Maintenance And Monitoring

Maintaining Health Habits

Maintaining excellent health practices is critical for long-term well-being, particularly for those with cervical cancer. It is not enough to make adjustments for a short period; you must also integrate them into your lifestyle over time. These habits apply to many elements of life, such as food, exercise, stress management, and so on. Consistency is essential for maintaining good health practices. Consistent adherence to a good diet, frequent physical exercise, efficient stress management, and enough rest are all essential components.

When it comes to nutrition, it's important to eat a range of nutrient-dense meals. This involves eating lots of fruits, veggies, whole grains, lean meats, and healthy fats. Diversifying your diet ensures that your body gets all of the vitamins, minerals, and antioxidants it needs to operate properly. Furthermore, staying hydrated by drinking lots of water throughout the day is critical to general health and well-being.

Regular exercise is another important component of sustaining healthy behaviors. Physical exercise not only helps with weight management, but it also improves mood, energy levels, and general quality of life. Aim for at least 30 minutes of moderate-intensity activity most days of the week, including activities you love like walking, swimming, or yoga.

Stress management strategies are also essential for long-term health. Chronic stress may damage the immune system, exacerbating cervical cancer symptoms. To relieve stress, use relaxation methods such as deep breathing, meditation, and mindfulness. Additionally, prioritize things that offer you pleasure and relaxation, such as spending time with loved ones, participating in hobbies, or appreciating nature.

The Need For Regular Check-Ups

Individuals with cervical cancer should have regular check-ups to maintain their health and spot any possible abnormalities early on. These check-ups may involve physical exams, blood tests, imaging studies, and other screenings to evaluate disease progression and look for indicators of recurrence. By being proactive about your health and scheduling frequent meetings with your healthcare practitioner, you may detect any changes or difficulties early on, when they are most curable.

In addition to screening for cancer-related issues, frequent check-ups enable healthcare experts to examine your general health and well-being. They may advise on how to live a healthy lifestyle, manage medication side effects, and handle any other health concerns that may develop. These sessions provide a chance to address any questions or concerns you may have regarding your health and treatment options.

Monitoring Nutritional Status

Monitoring your dietary condition is critical for treating cervical cancer and maintaining general health and well-being. Proper eating is crucial for maintaining strength, minimizing treatment side effects, and strengthening the immune system. It is critical to collaborate closely with a licensed dietitian or nutritionist to create a personalized nutrition plan based on your unique requirements and objectives.

Tracking your food consumption, monitoring weight and body composition changes, and checking blood work for vitamin shortages or imbalances are all examples of routine nutritional evaluations. Based on these evaluations, you may need to make dietary changes, such as boosting your calorie and protein consumption to promote healing and avoid muscle loss, or adopting particular foods to address nutritional shortages.

Adjusting Diet And Lifestyle As Needed

As your health demands change during your cancer treatment, you must be flexible and adaptive in your food and lifestyle choices. Certain treatments or drugs may alter your appetite, taste preferences, or digestion, necessitating dietary modifications to maintain proper nutrition and symptom control. Similarly, variations in physical activity or energy levels may need alterations to your workout regimen.

Stay in touch with your healthcare team and nutritionist to discuss any changes or issues you may be facing. They may provide advice and support as you manage these changes and make educated choices about your food and lifestyle. Remember that it is OK to seek assistance and support from loved ones or support groups during these times of transition.

Celebrating Progress & Milestones

Celebrating accomplishments and milestones during your cancer journey is critical for keeping motivation and a happy attitude. Whether it's reaching treatment milestones, attaining personal health objectives, or just persisting through difficult circumstances, acknowledging and celebrating these accomplishments may improve morale and offer a feeling of satisfaction.

Find methods to celebrate that are meaningful to you, such as treating yourself to a nice dinner, spending time with loved ones, or just reflecting and expressing thanks for how far you've gone. These celebrations serve as a reminder of your strength and perseverance in the face of hardship, allowing you to continue moving ahead with confidence and conviction.

Staying Up To Date On The Latest Research And Recommendations

Staying up to date on the latest cervical cancer research and guidelines is critical for making educated healthcare choices. Consult reliable sources such as medical publications, trusted websites, and healthcare specialists to stay current on advances in cancer therapy, supporting treatments, and lifestyle suggestions.

Talk with your healthcare provider about new research and treatment choices that may be relevant to your situation. Ask questions, seek clarification, and advocate for your needs to ensure you get the most up-to-date and effective treatment available. Consider joining support groups or online forums to interact with people going through similar issues and exchange knowledge and resources.

Staying informed and actively involved in your treatment allows you to make intelligent choices that benefit your health and well-being. Remember, information is power, and by being educated, you can actively manage your cervical cancer and live your best life.

CONCLUSION

The conclusion of cervical cancer nutrition emphasizes the importance of food and nutrition in the prevention and treatment of cervical cancer. A complete nutritional strategy may have a major influence on the overall health of those who are at risk of or have been diagnosed with cervical cancer.

For starters, a proper diet boosts the immune system, which is essential in the body's defense against human papillomavirus (HPV) infection, a leading cause of cervical cancer. Diets high in fruits, vegetables, whole grains, and lean meats include critical vitamins, minerals, and antioxidants that boost immune function and may lower the risk of HPV persistence and cancer development.

Second, some foods have been discovered as having possible preventive benefits against cervical cancer. Vitamins A, C, and E, as well as folate and carotenoids, have all been demonstrated to benefit cervical health. Incorporating meals rich in these nutrients may be advantageous. Furthermore, maintaining a healthy weight via balanced eating lowers the risk of chronic inflammation and hormone imbalances, both of which have been linked to cancer development.

Nutrition is essential for individuals receiving cervical cancer therapy to manage adverse effects and improve their quality of life. A well-planned diet may help patients manage symptoms including nausea, exhaustion, and weight loss, allowing them to retain their strength and energy levels. Tailored nutritional treatments may target particular requirements, such as increasing protein intake to promote tissue regeneration and giving enough calories to avoid malnutrition.

Finally, diet plays an important role in the comprehensive approach to cervical cancer prevention, treatment, and survival. Individuals who follow a nutrient-rich diet may strengthen their immune system, perhaps lessen their chance of getting cervical cancer, and enhance their response to therapy and general well-being. As part of comprehensive cervical cancer treatment, healthcare practitioners should emphasize the significance of nutrition and provide personalized nutritional advice.

THE END

9 798328 682022